To Madison, Shawna and Evelyn
you remind me to live every moment to the fullest,
and fill my heart with the love to live forever

To Andrew
It may not have played out as we'd expected,
but we still managed to make beautiful music

MAKE IT HAPPEN

SHOCK EVERY SINGLE ONE OF THEM

www.carlamjones.com

TABLE OF CONTENTS

DO SOMETHING TODAY THAT YOUR FUTURE SELF WILL THANK YOU FOR

Prologue

What if you could wake up tomorrow morning feeling the best you ever have? Imagine it for a second: no more fatigue, no more pains. You'd be vibrant with energy and motivation. You'd be HAPPY. HEALTHY. You'd be the person you always wanted to be...

What would be different? What would change? What would you do then, that you're not doing now? Would you climb Mount Kilimanjaro or hike the Appalachian trail? Would you quit an unsatisfying job and start an exciting career? Would you write a book or paint a masterpiece? Maybe, you'd finally be able to play with your kids and watch them get tired before you do?

We've all got goals. We all have things we'd like to do, and achieve. And almost every single person on this planet would like to feel healthier, more vibrant, more youthful and more beautiful. Don't you?

It's easy to look at those successful icons in our society and think that somehow, they were given something extra. Maybe they were blessed in some special way. Maybe they had people, things, money - everything required to succeed...

... or maybe, they were born a clean slate, just like you and me, and it is their lifestyle, their attitude and their energy that sets them apart.

But that means that if they're not special...

If their not special, then you have no excuses! If they can achieve their goals, then you can achieve yours. Simple, right? EXACTLY!

This simple guide is a 7 day stepping stone to eating better, sleeping better, living better and feeling better about yourself. On its own, it might not make you a multimillionaire, but it will set a foundation to health, acceptance and happiness... and that's a good place to start.

After you've completed these 7 days, you can purchase my "31 Days to a Healthier, Happier you" via my website, www.carlamjones.com, for an easy-to-follow month long plan to getting your nutrition and lifestyle on track for success. Then, sign up to my newsletter where I'll be divulging tips, recipes, inviting you to exclusive interviews with a variety of experts and programs to get you to target those behaviours and thought patterns that are holding you back and get you achieving all of your life's goals. It's just that easy! And I promise you - nothing could be more fun, or more rewarding than living the life you want.

How to use this book

This book was written with simplicity in mind. It's aimed at busy people who want to know what to do, but don't have the time to read long drawn out books filled with personal stories and other filler information. This book is clear cut, concise and gives you want you want: an easy to follow plan to get you living a healthier, happier life.

To maximise the effectiveness of this book, I recommend you read tomorrow's action plan today. This ensures that you are physically and mentally prepared for tomorrow's action step. There are 7 action steps. One for each day of this 1 week (7 day) program. Do these in the order they are written. They've been set in a particular order to maximise your potential to integrate them effortlessly into your day-to-day routine. We want to make small changes or tweaks to your daily habits. Smaller, more manageable actions makes it easier to achieve permanent changes. Keeping up with the action steps every day will create the foundation for a Healthier, Happier you.

As each day goes by, remember to keep doing the actions of previous days. There is a cumulative effect to this program. Some will be dietary changes, some will be lifestyle habits... some will happen only in your mind. All are easily achievable by anyone who reads this.

So... go on... let's not drag this on any further. A Healthier, Happier YOU awaits!

** A special thank you **

If you've decided to download "7 Days to a Healthier, Happier You", I thank you. My quest to making this world a healthier and happier place for my children to live in starts with you! As a Thank you, I'd like to offer you a FREE 30-min Wellness Strategy Session. It will allow you to speak to me directly about the things you've tried, the goals you want to achieve and how we can start you on your personalised successful Wellness Plan. Your wellness includes your diet, your body, your lifestyle... your goals for any aspect of your life that will make you happier, so don't be shy, book today:

https://carlamjones.acuityscheduling.com

Making it Work

If you can't fly, then run
If you can't run, then walk
If you can't walk, then crawl
but whatever you do,
you have to keep moving forward.

- Martin Luther King Jr.

www.carlamjones.com

Tips and Strategies to achieving permanent changes

Making permanent changes in our life is probably one of the hardest things anyone can do. But all hope is not lost. Making changes IS possible! The following are some tips and strategies to making permanent changes possible for YOU and making it an easy task to succeed!

- **Visualize:** You've decided to make changes in your life. You want to feel better, get more energy, live an enviable life… That's great! What does this mean to you? Close your eyes for 2mins and paint a mental picture of what this means to you. What does it look like? What does it smell like? What sounds are you hearing? How will you feel when you succeed? What will you do then that you're not doing now? The more detail you can put into your mental image of what you're after, the more power your visualisation will have to remind you, in times of need, of the reason you've decided to make this change. When you're struggling with your new habits, take 30secs and bring back that *image of success, your visualisation* - it's a great form of inspiration.
- **Be Mentally prepared:** Read tomorrow's action, today… so you know what you have to do. This will allow you to become mentally prepared for it, and ensure you have all of the tools (and none of the excuses) to get it done.
- **Start your day with a plan:** know what change you are going to make, and take 3mins when you wake up and tell yourself: "Today, I AM *making this change"* Remember to stay positive. Your subconscious will remember to keep you on track

if you state changes in the present, as if the change is already being done.

- **Start small:** that drive you're feeling to change will last longer if you start with small manageable changes. Remember this is a marathon (not a sprint)... so no matter how quickly you want to overhaul your life, *Walk - don't run* to your destination.

- **Create a tracking sheet:** This can be a visual tracking sheet on the refrigerator or an alert that pops up on your smartphone. It doesn't matter how you prefer to be reminded - put the right systems in place to be reminded every time you have a new habit (action) to do... and then *do it!* (A Tracking sheet for week 1 is available in the Appendix).

- **Keep it visible:** Part of keeping a tracking sheet is the benefit of having it as a visible reminder. Remember the age-old saying: "Out of sight, Out of mind..." so keep a reminder of your new habit (action) visible until doing it has become second nature (Studies show that it takes on average 21 days to adopt a new habit, but it takes between 66 days for our brain to create the neural pathways to make that habit sub-consciously permanent).

- **If you fall off the horse, don't dwell:** just get back on that horse and keep going. The longer you've been doing a particular habit, the harder it will be to change it. Time, life, cravings... these are all things that can get in the way of a particular new habit on a specific occasion. If you forget a new habit one time, don't dwell. It's OK. Just get back to the new habit as quickly as possible and keep going.

- **Seek support:** The best way to stay on track is to get others to support you. Find a friend to make the change with you or hire a coach who will create a plan specifically designed for you, support you with the challenges and cheer your successes. Check out **www.carlamjones.com** for Nutrition, Health and Wellness Coaching programs.

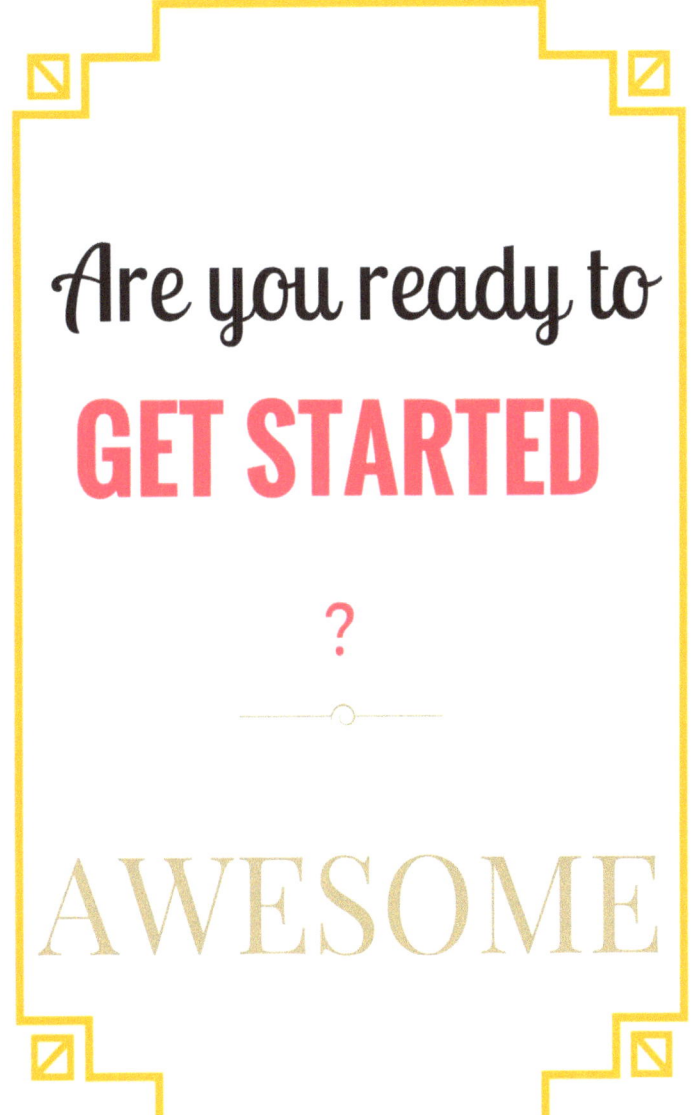

Are you ready to

GET STARTED

?

AWESOME

Tasty Hydration

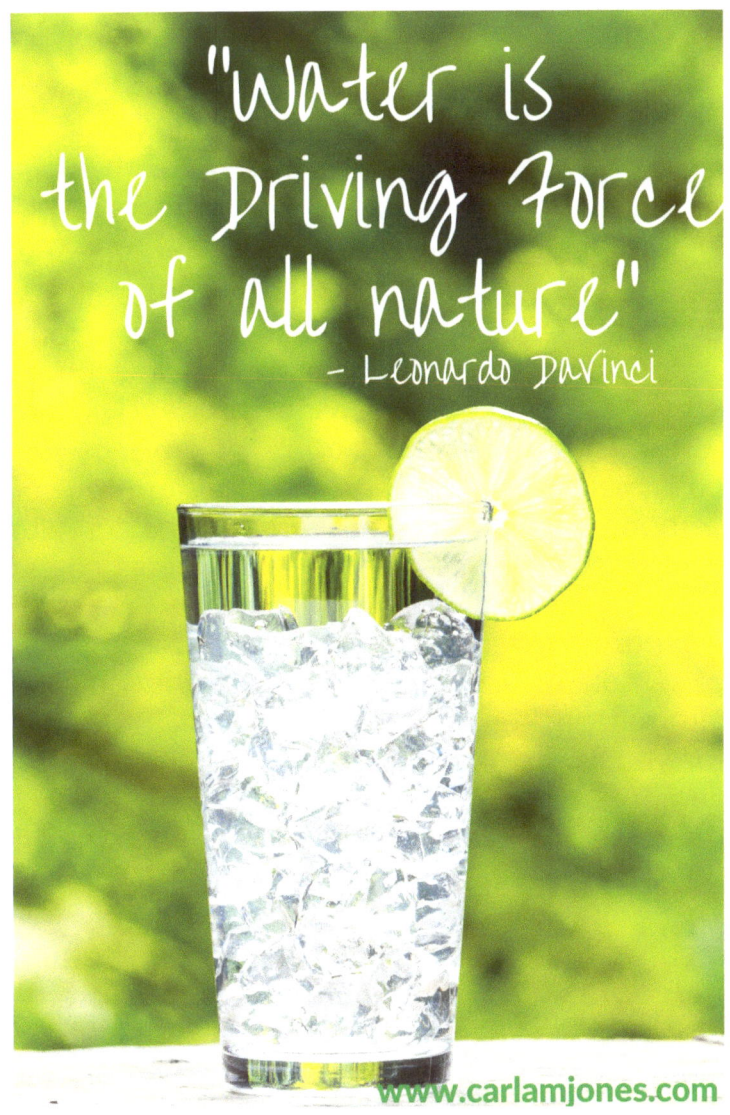

"Water is the Driving Force of all nature"
- Leonardo DaVinci

www.carlamjones.com

When you wake up in the morning, do you feel more like a force of nature or the aftermath of a big storm?

If you feel sluggish and reluctant to get up, in the morning, and you find that constant energy during the day is one of your biggest challenges, the solution may be as simple as a glass of water.

Starting the morning with a warm glass of lemon water has many benefits. Here are just a few:

1. Lemons are bright yellow and smell great. Yellow fruits and vegetables are generally **high in Bioflavanoids, Carotenoids and Vitamin C**, all of which are responsible for improving overall health. It might be all the vitamins and hydrating electrolytes available to us from the lemon, or maybe, it's that tart citric aroma that gets you going, but starting the day with lemon water is an **instant boost of energy** to the body, and a great substitute to a morning coffee.
2. Lemons are jam packed with vitamin C. Vitamin C is important to keep us fighting off colds and flus by **boosting our immune system**. Flavouring your water with the juice of 1/4 - 1/2 of lemon means that you start the day with a vitamin packed drink that is delicious and good for you.
3. Lemons *promote good digestion* thanks to their pectin levels. Pectin is a soluble fibre. Soluble fibre dissolves in water to form a gel. This gel slows down the digestion process which means your body has *more time to absorb valuable vitamins and nutrients* from the foods you eat, and as a bonus, you feel fuller for longer, experience less hunger cravings, making

you less likely to snack. This is helpful in controlling **weight** and **stabilising blood sugar levels.** Soluble fibres, such as pectin, have also been known to **reduce LDL ("bad") cholesterol.**

4. The Vitamin C in lemons **may also improve your skin**. Vitamin C helps the body to produce Collagen. Collagen keeps our skin firm and slows down the ageing of our skin.

MAKING IT HAPPEN

The best way to make sure you start your day with lemon water is to have everything pre-ready. Pre-cut your lemons the night before and place them in the fridge in an airtight container. This ensures minimal prep in the morning and prevents any injuries from using a sharp knife when you're still groggy and half asleep.

Squeeze the lemon into a glass, then fill it up with room temperature water. If you can warm up the water in a kettle for 1 - 2 min, the lemon water will be more easily absorbed into your body.

Routine is very important in creating new habits so, decide on where this habit fits into your already set morning routine, and repeat it in the same manner every morning. And remember that easing into habits is a better way to sticking with them:

- start by drinking water for a few days.
- once this starts to feel natural, add the juice of 1/4 lemon
- after a few days, add the juice of 1/2 lemon

WORTH MENTIONING

Warm is best in the morning, and if you like the flavour, lemon water is great all day long. 1 glass, 30mins before each meal helps get the stomach acids ready to digest your meals, curbs hunger, and keeps you hydrated.

De-Electromagnetify

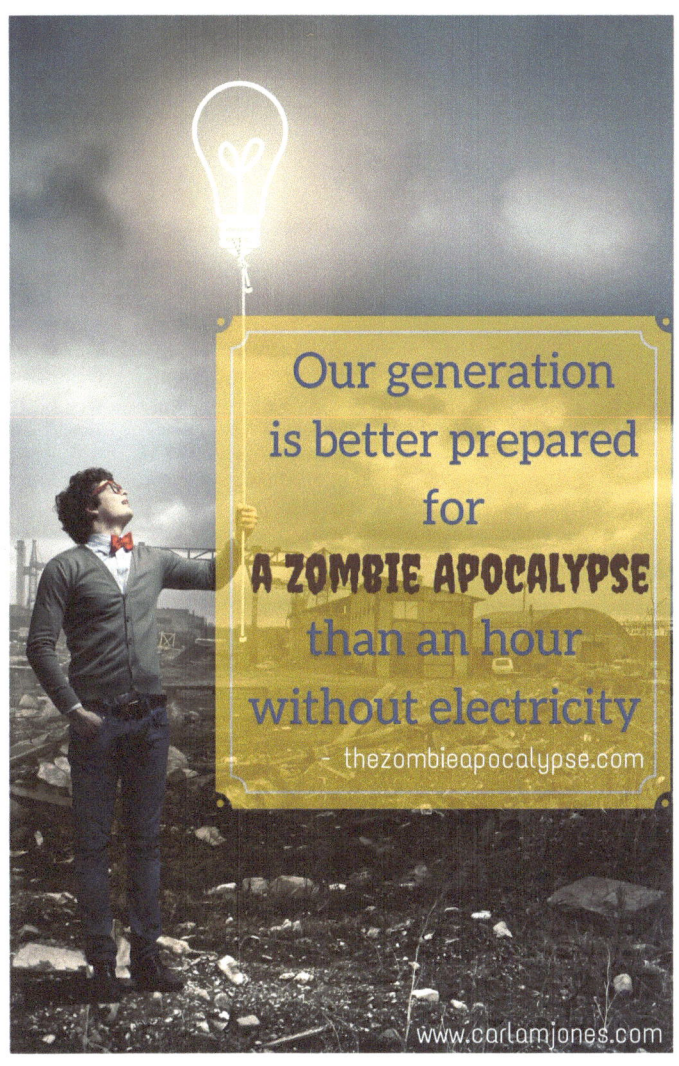

Our generation is better prepared for **A ZOMBIE APOCALYPSE** than an hour without electricity

- thezombieapocalypse.com

www.carlamjones.com

OK, so "de-electromagnetify" is not a real word - you won't find it in any dictionary. But it is a good way to remember that you must release the Electro Magnetic energy being built up in your body all day long by devices that release electromagnetic energy. These devices include the TV, your computer, your laptop, your tablet and your smartphone... Do any of these go to bed with you?

As a society, we are constantly being "charged" with electro magnetic energy. That energy builds up in our bodies. Everything in the world needs a resting period: summer turns into winter, day turns into night... and our bodies need to sleep - soundly and deeply, to regenerate.

When we sleep, we transition between REM and Non-REM Sleep. Our body dreams, assimilates information from the day and heals & repairs itself from the wears and tears of everyday life. Our body requires approximately 8 consecutive hours of sleep because our sleep cycles have a natural rhythm and it is vitally important to go through all of the proper stages of sleep in order to benefit from them.

Electronic devices (as well as artificial lighting) disrupt our sleep patterns because it keeps our bodies in a "charged" mode. Altering our natural sleep cycle, this way, means that our bodies keep producing daytime hormones instead of nighttime ones (like melatonin, which make us sleepy). This has a domino effect on lots of other body functions, which can have negative effects on our stages of sleep patterns and their ability to heal and restore our bodies.

In fact, studies show that insufficient quality sleep can lead to depression, hormonal issues, digestive problems and metabolic syndrome (a group of risk factors such as high blood pressure, high cholesterol, and high blood sugar, which then can lead to a variety of diseases).

MAKING IT HAPPEN

It is quite simple, really: turn off all electronic devices at least 30 mins (but preferably 60mins) before going to sleep. And if you turn off the lights before bedtime, or at least keep them very dim, this will help you sleep better as well.

SO WHAT DO I DO INSTEAD?

In our busy world of emails, social media, endless addictive apps and 24hr-on demand viewing, it's easy to forget to be human beings, again. So, here is a short list to get you started on filling the time before bed with non-electronic-dependent activities:

- read a good *paper* book
- tidy up
- walk the dog
- talk to your spouse about *their* dreams
- write a bucket list for your life
- make love
- take a bath
- write your memoirs
- pray
- give thanks
- meditate
- keep a journal
- play a board game, dominos, or cards
- work off your day's energy by making dough, kneading it with all your might for at least 20

mins, then let it rise overnight to find a wholesome gift of yumminess waiting to be baked in the morning for a gorgeous breakfast treat: **homemade bread!** (see Appendix for a suggested recipe)

This list is by no means extensive and you can let your creativity take over. If you can't think of anything to do, just ask yourself: "What would my grandparents have done before bedtime?" And you've got your answer!

Take the BMW

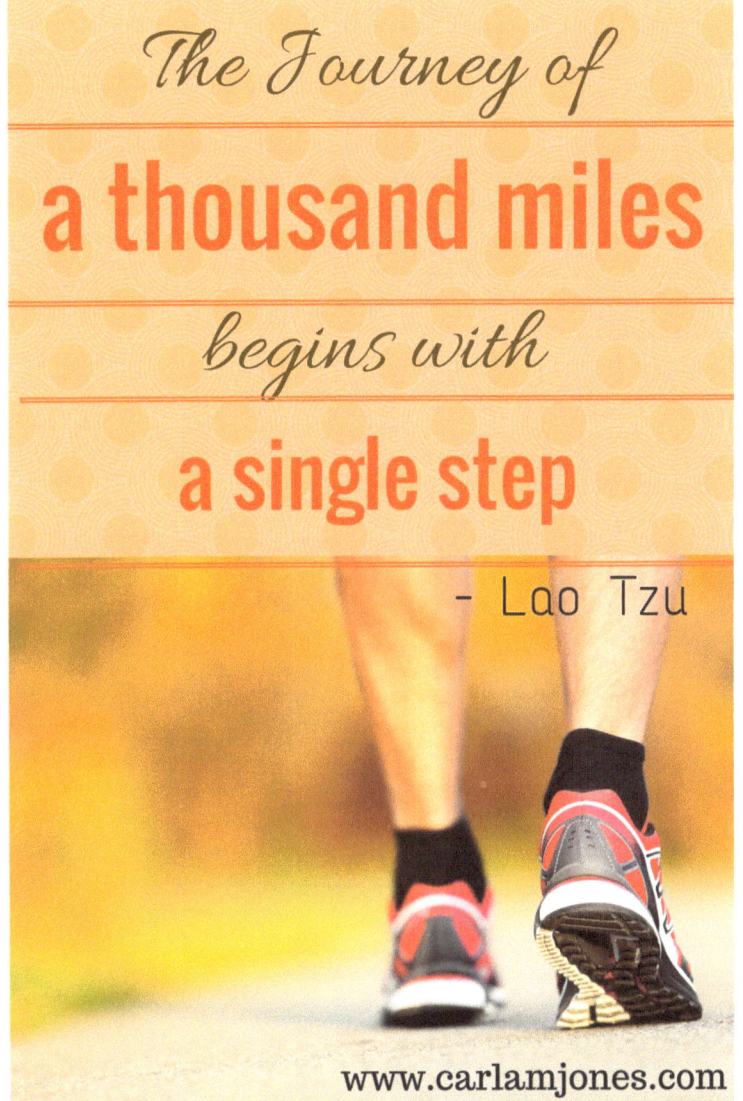

The Journey of **a thousand miles** begins with **a single step**

\- Lao Tzu

www.carlamjones.com

No! this is not a sponsored ad for a car manufacturer. In this case, I am referring to taking a mode of transportation that most of us have forgotten still exists: **B**us, **M**etro (subway), **W**alk... or in other words - Your FEET!

That's right! Your Feet are a great way to get around: they allow us to see everything at a pace that works for us. They allow us to stop easily, where ever we want, to smell the roses, say 'hello' to a friend or grab a coffee and a book and watch the world go by. More impressively, using our feet to get where we need to go allows us to increase our activity level, our heart rate and our levels of happiness (thank you endorphins)... and it's a great way to de-compress, clear some headspace and think creatively! Not bad for an absolutely FREE activity!

 ARE YOU KEEPING UP?

Increasing your activity level also increases your body's need for water as it dehydrates through sweating.

Extra hydration is important, in particular, on days with increased activity.

You can re-read ~Day 1~ if you have doubts about how to hydrate properly and deliciously.

Now, I'm not suggesting you start walking marathon lengths to get to work everyday. I am suggesting that whenever there is the alternative to walk - You take it! Walk to the park, walk to the convenience store, walk around the block or walk the dog a little extra everyday. The key, here, is to

WALK! As often as possible, walk briskly and for a minimum of 20mins. If you can do it daily, great! If you can do it 3 times a week, that's good too! The important thing is to add it into your schedule and keep at it.

MAKING IT HAPPEN

Not sure if you're walking enough? Download an app to your smartphone and keep your phone with you on your walks: it'll calculate the number of steps you take a day (and you should be aiming for at least 10,000 steps). If you work at a desk, drive to work, and you don't go to the gym... you're probably averaging about 1,000 steps a day... so Start Walking!!!

Another great way to make sure you're walking enough is to start a lunchtime walking group with work colleagues or neighbourhood friends (having a support system is always a great way to take up a new activity). Can't find anyone to walk with? That's ok! Most smartphone activity apps will connect you with people around the world to keep you accountable, and challenge you to the next level of activity.

Another alternative is to ditch the car and take public transport: you'll have to walk to the bus stop or subway station, go up and down the stairs (take the active option instead of the escalator, please), then walk to wherever it is your

going (and then do it all again on your way back home). You can start this once a week to work, and slowly increase it over time. And if you're lucky enough to live close to work, another great alternative is to cycle! (And "bike-to-work" tax incentives and programs are becoming a very popular thing in major cities around the world, so find out with your city council if such a program is in place where you live).

WORTH MENTIONING

We're looking for ways to naturally increase your activity level on a daily basis, without increasing the costs. Walking is a low intensity / high reward activity. It is a great way to start. If you can't walk, find another physical activity to keep active. Aim to raise your heart rate for at least 20mins a day, 3 times a week.

Go old-skool

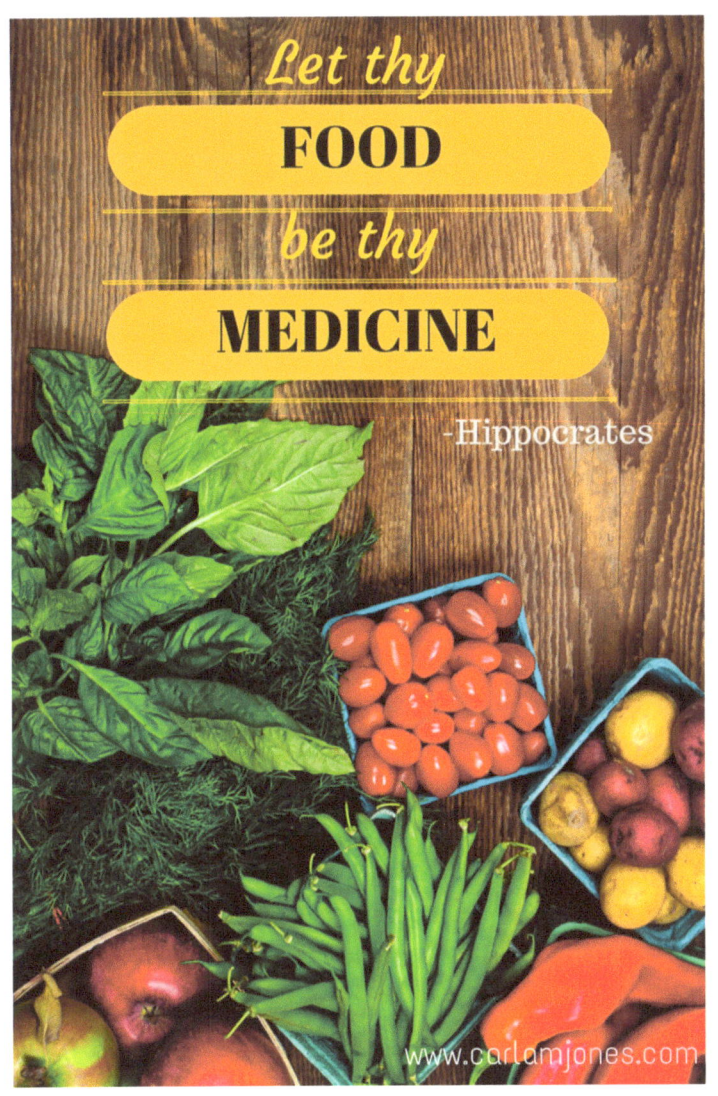

According to the World Health Organization, in 2005, chronic diseases accounted for over 60% of all deaths around the world. The WHO considers this to be an epidemic that is silently taking over the world. In a 2010 survey, it was found that over 50% of the population surveyed around the world were Obese or Overweight. This ratio jumped to a staggering 65% of the population when looking at just the Americas, Australia, and the more developed parts of Europe and Africa.

A Chronic Disease is an illness that is non-communicable (non-contagious) and can be influenced by lifestyle. As a result, Chronic Diseases are sometimes labelled "Lifestyle Diseases". Their effects are long lasting and progress slowly. The most common of these diseases are Cardiovascular (ex: heart attacks and strokes), certain Cancers, Chronic Respiratory Diseases (ex: Asthma) and Diabetes.

All of these are greatly determined by your diet and lifestyle. Here is a quick survey to determine whether you need to change your diet:

- Do you eat in restaurants or take-away food more than 1x per week?
- Do you eat pre-packaged foods (fish fingers, chicken nuggets, frozen lasagnas, sauces in a jar, store-bought salad dressings...)?
- Do you eat processed foods (white bread, white sugar, breakfast cereals, soft drinks or energy drinks, store-bought juices)?
- Do you feel energy slumps mid-morning and/or mid-afternoon?
- Is Beige the primary colour of the food you eat?

If you answered YES to the questions above, then you are not eating a "whole food diet", and your body is not taking advantage of all of the healing, healthy benefits you can get from the foods you eat in their natural form.

In a nutshell, we can all agree that nature is perfect! Everything was created with a purpose. For example, eating an apple a day provides you with an array of vitamins that may, in fact, keep the doctor away. If you're eating the pips, than you are also ingesting small amounts of cyanide - which is a lethal poison. However, nature, in its infinite perfection, has coated the apple seeds with a husk that is hard to chew, and difficult to digest in order to protect us from the poison inside. See? Perfect!

In its perfection, nature has given us a wide range of foods to eat to ensure our body gets everything it needs to live a healthy strong life. An abundance of colours to choose from in the produce section allows us to visually replenish our diet with a rainbow of vitamins and nutrients essential to our health. But there is a caveat: we have to stick to whole foods! In other words, we have to stick to eating foods as close to their natural state as possible, in order to benefit from what nature has to give us. Overcooking our foods or altering them with industrial processes turns all of our food to Beige - and Beige has no nutritional value.

To make it easier on us, we can use nature's cheat sheet: a colour-coded system to identifying the primary phytonutrients and vitamins available in the produce we eat. Not only does this make our task of eating healthy whole foods easy - it also makes our dinner plate a beautiful colour-rich work of culinary art, provided to us by nature, for our wellbeing. And of course, the more colour you add to your plate, the more benefits you are getting.

Easy right? It couldn't be any simpler - or more delicious than this! You can find Nature's cheat sheet in the Appendix.

MAKING IT HAPPEN

If you're not sure you are eating a Whole Food diet, ask yourself this one question:

Was this food available to my grandparents when they were growing up?

It may sound like a silly question to ask yourself, but if you think about it… so many of the world's health issues can be traced back to our increasingly poor diet, made up of quick, easy and inexpensive foods. Frozen foods, breaded foods, highly processed meals, industrial preservatives, food colourings and additives, anything from a vending machine… these were not available to our grandparents when they were growing up. Industrial foods may be cheaper at the till, but the true price tag comes much later, and costs us our health.

Going Old-skool - in other words, back to our ancestral way of eating may save us from a wide range of lifestyle illnesses. More fresh fruit and vegetables (more colour) and less processed foods (beige) will make your plate more visually appealing and healthier. And the natural benefits given to us by nature are a gift that our future self will thank us for.

D-minish D-ficiency

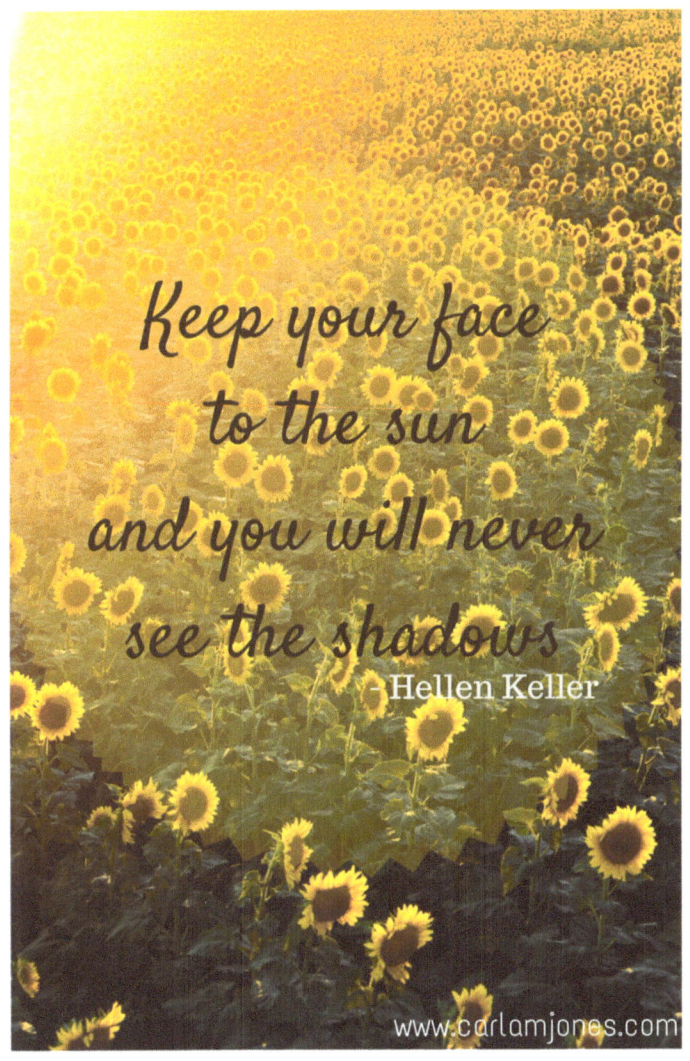

Keep your face
to the sun
and you will never
see the shadows
- Hellen Keller

www.carlamjones.com

Each day of this book has had an angle. You've either been making a little change in your diet or your lifestyle or your mind (Day 7's action).

Today, you are achieving a change that affects your diet, lifestyle and mind. This kind of action is like buying 1 and getting 2 more for free. It's like getting what you want in one fell swoop.

What does it involve? Getting more Vitamin D.

This might sound like a fairly simple task to do. Take a vitamin and Bam! Bob's your uncle. But not all Vitamin D is the same and knowing the difference can save you loads on supplements.

For starters, let's quickly review Vitamin D - what is it? where do you get it? What's it good for?

Vitamin D is an unusual vitamin. Our biggest source of Vitamin D does not come from food. It is synthesised from Cholesterol when our skin is exposed to the sun. (D3 - cholecalciferol). We can also find some amounts of Vitamin D in certain foods such as mushrooms and salmon. This type of Vitamin D is called ergocalciferol or Vitamin D2. It was once believed that Vitamin D was a fat-soluble vitamin necessary for Healthy Bones. Now we know that it is also a hormone that helps to regulate our metabolism, allowing it to function properly. Vitamin D has been discovered to be essential is such metabolic functions such as:

- maintaining stable levels of calcium in our blood and tissues
- maintaining bone density and strength in adults (and proper bone development in children)

- regulating cell development - particularly white blood cells (immune system) and epithelial cells (good skin)
- strengthening the immune system
- regulating insulin activity
- regulating blood sugar balance
- regulating blood pressure
- maintaining muscle function
- staving off Seasonal Affective Disorder (SAD) - a type of depression occurring in dark winter month

The sources of vitamin D are limited. The best source is from the sun on your bare skin (D3 - Cholecalciferol). But some foods also naturally contain Vitamin D (D2 - ergocalciferol) such as : Full fat Dairy produce, Oily fish, Cod liver oil, Salmon, Tuna (fresh not canned), Shrimp, Sunflower seeds, Liver, Egg yolks and Mushrooms. Additionally, you'll also find many Vitamin D fortified foods on the market today such as bread and milk.

Despite sunny summer months and many outdoor activities to choose from, many of us are Vitamin D deficient. This is often due to the use of sunblocks such as lotions, makeup and moisturisers that come with an SPF grade. Sun blocking creams prohibit the necessary UV rays from penetrating the skin, and therefore, prevent any Vitamin D from being absorbed or metabolised in the body. Though the use of sunblock is advisable and recommended in the prevention of burns and skin cancers, it is worth while spending a little time "unprotected" to ensure your body's been topped up with Vitamin D.

MAKING IT HAPPEN

Whenever possible, stand in the sun and face it, eyes closed, for 10 - 15 mins. (you can put on the sunscreen after the 15mins, and for the rest of the day). This will allow your body to absorb Vitamin D3 and synthesise it effectively. If it's winter, or you live in a non-sunny place, review the list of food sources above, and add them into your meal plan every week, as often as possible.

WORTH MENTIONING

If you're thinking of buying a vitamin D supplement, it is important to read the label to find out the source (look for whole food sources - not chemical/pharmaceutical creations) and aim to find a D3 (Cholecalciferol) supplement. Taking a supplement that has been created from a natural source may make the supplement more expensive, but it will be easier for your body to absorb and metabolise what it needs.

Brainiac Breakfasts

"When you wake up in the morning, Pooh,"
said Piglet at last

"What's the first thing you say to yourself?
"What's for Breakfast?"
said Pooh.

"What do you say, Piglet?"
"I say, I wonder what's going to happen exciting today?"
said Piglet

Pooh nodded thoughtfully...
"It's the same thing."

- Winnie the Pooh

www.carlamjones.com

Does this sound like you?

- Wake-up
- Take a shower
- Get dressed
- Have a quick coffee
- Head to work/drop off kids at school
- Grab a muffin, bowl of cereal, or piece of fruit to eat on the way
- Get to work (or back home)
- Work
- Feel sluggish mid-morning
- Grab another coffee and quick (sweet/salty) snack
- Back to work
- Starving by lunch
- Grab a quick lunch - maybe a Chef's salad or Sandwich or Soup (because you're trying to be healthy / lose weight)
- Back to work
- Feeling tired mid-afternoon
- Grab another coffee
- Head home (impatient with other drivers)
- Impatient with kids
- Prepare dinner
- Eat
- Grab a sweet treat or salty snack while watching TV
- Bed

You're not alone! Today's action is to start eating a healthy, protein-rich breakfast - within 1 hour of waking up!

It's a pretty precise action, and this one may take some getting used to day-to-day. But it is one of the most important things you can do to improve your memory and concentration, improve your mood, improve your level of patience, feel energetic, reduce energy slumps and cut back on coffee or other stimulants.

Not bad for just 1 action step!

Why is a protein-rich breakfast so important?

Protein is one of the essential macronutrients required for our body to operate efficiently. Protein makes up approximately 18% of our total body mass. We use it to provide us with energy, build and maintain muscle, and to regulate a wide variety of body functions such as the acidity/alkalinity of our bodies, hormone levels and blood sugar levels.

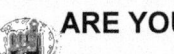 **ARE YOU KEEPING UP?**

If you've been following all of the steps and integrating them into your day-to-day life, you have made huge efforts in achieving a healthier, happier you.

Congratulations!

Only one more day to go!! These actions should become routine in no time. Just keep at it, and you'll get there! I believe in you and your infinite power to lead the life you want!

A healthy human adult will make and use approximately 300gr of protein each day. So, replenishing the protein stocks in our body is vital to the proper functioning of our body.

Eating breakfast within an hour of waking up gives your body the fuel it needs when you wake up. Even if you tend to have something to eat before bedtime, by the time you wake up in the morning, you've gone at least 6-9 hours without eating. If you wait until mid-morning to have something to eat (or until lunchtime), your body enters into starvation mode and is more likely to store more of what you eat (the good and the bad) rather than flushing out what it doesn't need. This is a biological instinct that dates back to our hunter gatherer years where humans were more likely to eat in a Feast or Famine situation. Storing energy reserves for a period of "famine" helped our survival back then. Now, this same bodily instinct promotes weight gain and needs to be maintained in a way that suits our modern life.

One of the most important roles of Protein in our diet is in regulating blood sugars. Blood sugars affect our body's production and resistance to insulin. When insulin is being poorly managed over a long period of time, it can lead to Diabetes, who's prevalence is one of the fastest growing chronic diseases in the world. Regulating blood sugars also has a myriad of secondary effects such as improved concentration, hormonal balancing (making you happier and more patient), and keeping energy levels up in the daytime.

Ensuring your breakfast is rich in protein helps to stabilise blood sugars throughout the day, by slowing down the digestion of carbohydrates. A slower digestion process means you'll feel fuller for longer, which in turn means less cravings for sweet and salty snacks. It also means your body has more time to absorb the good vitamins and nutrients from the food you eat. This is all good news if you are working on weight maintenance or weight loss.

You can find a list of easy to make Protein-rich breakfast ideas in the Appendix.

WORTH MENTIONING

It's important to note that Protein should only account for approximately 20-25% of your diet (Dietary Fats and Carbohydrates making up the other 75-80%). Protein deficiency has its consequences, but the over-consumption of protein is equally detrimental to our wellbeing.

Additionally, not all protein is the same. A protein shake or bar is often loaded in sugars, preservatives, and food additives. Though they have their uses in certain situations, this is not a healthy way to get your daily protein intake (especially at breakfast) and they should never be used to replace a well-balanced diet. When choosing a source of protein, aim for the highest quality you can afford. Good quality proteins include: lean chicken breast, whole eggs, lentils, tuna, quinoa, wheat germ, lean beef, millet, cottage cheese, and nuts.

Kill the Gremlin

Everytime you think

I can't do this

**You've already
decided
the outcome**

www.carlamjones.com

When we are born, we are a like an empty clean jar. We have no judgement, no opinions, no beliefs, no values. We are free. Free to achieve anything. Free to be anything. Everyone loves babies because babies remind us of all of the good in the world. Babies represent possibilities - dreams - achievement. No one ever looks at a baby and thinks: "this one will amount to nothing". We look at a baby and think: "Future president" "Future Nobel winner" "Future *enter-your-dream-of-success-here*". Parents often promise to protect their child, care and nurture that child no matter what. The child WILL BE the very best it can be.

Something strange happens as we grow up. Our empty clean jar becomes filled with thoughts and ideas and opinions. We start filling our jar of possibilities with post-it notes, reminders and pictures of fear, anger, missed opportunities, wrong decisions, have-nots and doubts. Worse even, we start to fill that jar with the opinions, fear, anger, missed opportunities, wrong decisions, have-nots and doubts of the people around us. Unwillingly, those who swore to protect us when we were babies, have their own battles to fight, and have a hard time keeping their own fears from affect our vision of the world. Our jar becomes full of negative notes and pictures. It becomes dirty and loses it's sparkle. Soon, the possibilities become harder to see through the murky glass and everything around us seems impossible, unachievable, not meant for us.

Most people will know what this feels like. Carrying doubt and fear and the feeling that we are moving slowly through life because of this heavy jar of negativity and impossibilities that we drag around.

This load holds us back and talks to us all the time. It picks up a "friend" along the way to help bare the weight. This "friend" talks to us in the first person and says things like:

- I can't do this;
- I'm too old for this;
- I'm not good enough because I never graduated;
- I'm so stupid;
- I'm such a klutz;
- If I do this, everyone will laugh.

Does any of this sound familiar?

This "friend" is a Gremlin that sits inside our head. It lives there because we've given it free room and board. It's there because every time it speaks to us, we feed it by listening to it and doing exactly what it wants. This Gremlin is the opposite of that cute little baby full of possibilities. It is a shrivelled up little monster with nasty teeth and foul breath, who slobbers all over our shoulder every time we give in to our fears and anger and doubt.

Do you want to kill the Gremlin?

Killing the Gremlin is a lot easier than you would think. There is only one weapon in the whole world that can manage such a task. This weapon is free and becomes stronger and more effective each time you use it. This weapon is:

Love

MAKE IT HAPPEN

This could be a whole book in itself.. and maybe a thought for future consideration. Until that book is written, here is a quick 7 step guide on *How to Kill the Gremlin Dead in its Tracks*

1. Acknowledge the negative self-talk. Once you've learned to recognise the Gremlin, he'll be easier to spot every time he wants to show himself. Recognising the Gremlin means you can stop him before he's had a chance to influence you.
2. Not sure your thoughts are Gremlin talk? Imagine hearing a 5 year old speaking your thoughts. What would you do? Would you let them keep up the talk or would you intervene and change their thoughts into something more positive, more inspiring, more forgiving... If it's not good enough for a 5 year old - it's not good enough for you
3. Forgive Forgive Forgive. Yourself, others, the world. No one is perfect and we all make mistakes. It's OK. Making mistakes means there was something to learn - and learning something new, even if only to make sure it doesn't happen again, is a blessing!
4. Understand the root Where does your negative self-talk come from. Is it fear? Is it Anger? It is something someone told you over and over when you were growing up? Understanding the root cause of your Gremlin talk means you can fight it head on: imagine yourself doing exactly what you want. Imagine yourself doing it well and being a big success at it. Imagine what it feels like, smells like, tastes like, and sounds like. Keep

imagining it, with as much detail as possible, until thinking about all that good drowns out the Gremlin.

5. Find an inspiration We all need role-models in life, and in the age of information, there are many to choose from. Find someone who's background, life and challenges resemble yours. Read up on them. Find out how they overcame their Gremlin - then use their experience to guide you.

6. Keep a journal Journaling your thoughts is a great way to become aware of yourself, and work through anything that is holding you back. Whenever you enter a Gremlin challenge, turn it around and find the positive. Be the 5 year old. Think or say inspirational thoughts to yourself. "I can do this because I can do anything I set my mind to".

7. Meditate with affirmations Every morning, take 5 mins to breathe. It should be a quiet place where you'll be undisturbed. Breathe deeply as you imagine your air coming from deep inside your belly and out your mouth. In with the nose, out with the mouth. Inhale for 4 seconds, hold your breath for 4 seconds, exhale slowly as long as it takes. When you're holding your breath, think positive thoughts:

- I am confident and strong
- I love and accept myself
- I am capable of anything I set my mind to
- I am special and unique
- I have many gifts that only I can bring into this world
- I am amazing

Killing the Gremlin won't happen overnight - that little monster has been fighting for his survival your whole life. But keep hitting him on the head with love... Lots of love... All of the love you have for yourself... and he'll eventually disappear for good.

Kill the Gremlin - Love yourself

Be Healthy and Nutritionally WELL-thy.

Carla M. Jones

About the Author

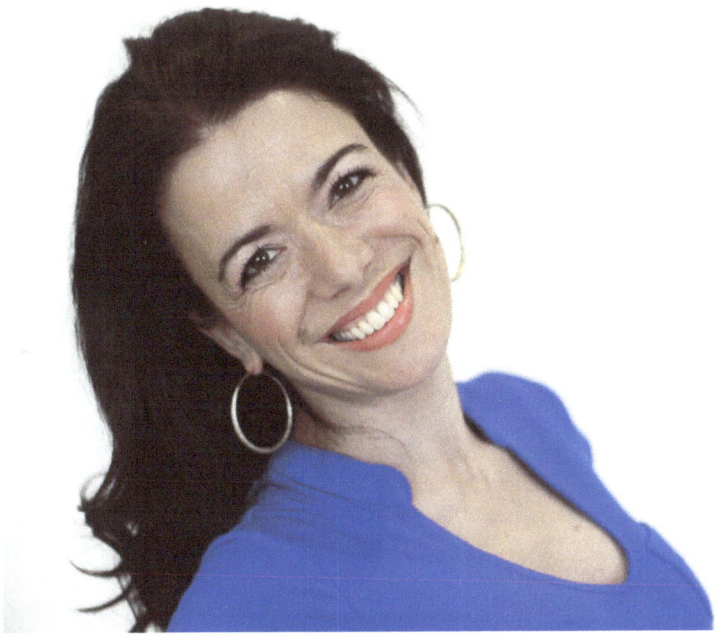

Ex-Marketing Director in the IT industry, Carla woke up one day and realised that she needed to return to her creative passions.

Giving up career, income and status, Carla returned to school despite all of the financial and family responsibilities on her plate. Now, Carla is living a purpose driven life where she gets to do what she loves and helps others achieve their own health and life goals, as well.

Carla is a well rounded Chef, Sommelier and Nutrition, Health & Wellness Coach, certified in the world's top Culinary and Nutrition schools. Additionally she is also a certified NLP practitioner and Stress Management counsellor. Carla's array of professional experience spans the globe. This includes, 4-star hotels and top restaurants across Asia and North America; running her own catering company in Spain; hosting a popular TV Cooking show on the Spanish food network; and currently, teaching and running a web-based Nutrition and Wellness clinic out of Dublin, Ireland.

One of Carla's deepest beliefs is that life should be fun. Her positive attitude and go-getter curiosity fuels the way she lives, teaches and experiences the world around her. Food is the medium by which she encourages others to explore happiness - ensuring that every recipe has been created to energise, 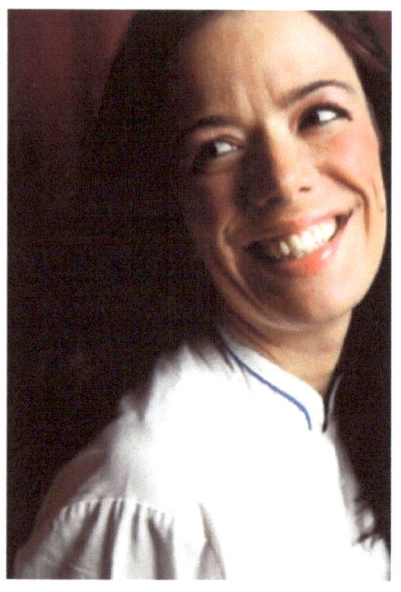 balance and encourage optimal health. Carla's passion comes across whenever she talks about food. She has the ability to make everything easy and achievable: from impossible techniques in the kitchen to picking up new habits in our lives. Carla's business is driven by her strong conviction that healthy eating and living is possible for everyone to achieve, regardless of budget, time or experience in the kitchen. Her enthusiasm for healthy, happy living quickly infects those around her and pushes them to achieve great results in their own lives.

Behind the scenes, Carla is a busy mom of 3 little girls and fully understands the constraints that people have when it comes to feeding their family.

Carla's daughters have learned that eating well means more health, more happiness and more energy to have fun. Among their favourite things to eat are Broccoli, Brussels sprouts and even Kale. Focused on healthy fun food for even the littlest tummy in the house, Carla's kids are always in the kitchen learning, tasting and experiencing food beside her. Carla's daughters remind her that it's never too late to learn about health and never too soon to teach our children how to eat healthy.

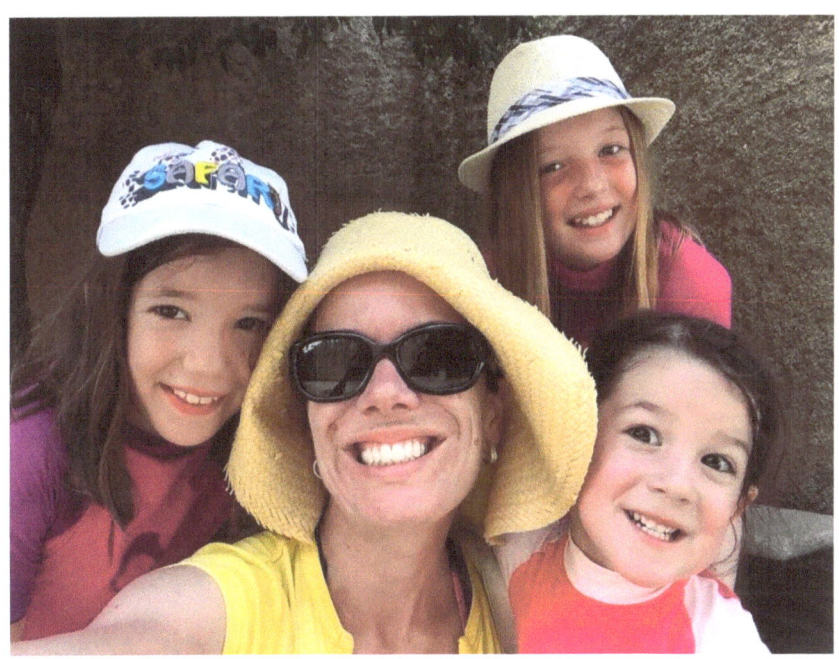

Appendix

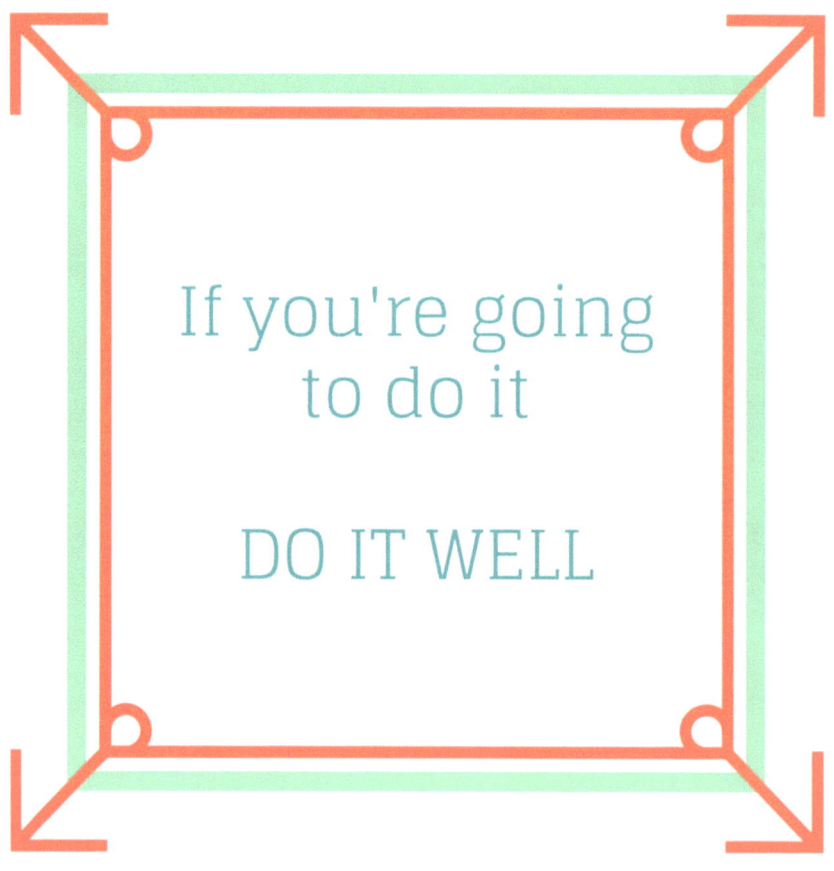

If you're going
to do it

DO IT WELL

Congratulations! You've completed small and manageable changes over the last 7 days that will build a foundation of health and happiness for years to come.

It is up to you to keep it up. Are you up for the challenge? The rewards are immeasurable!

As mentioned previously in this book, making permanent changes takes time, thought (reminders) and motivation. These initial changes are quick and easy additions to your daily routine. If you enjoyed these past 7 days, you are encouraged to gather a group of friends and continue this program together (having a buddy keeps up the motivation and helps you stay accountable to your actions). My complete "31 days to a Healthier, Happier you" program will be available soon, so, make sure to sign-up to the newsletter for updates, links and promotions.

Over the following pages, you will find some additional resources to help you get the most out of this book.

- **7 Day Tracking sheet**
     - Post this onto your refrigerator, bathroom mirror or office. This is your visual reminder to stay on track, this first week.
- **Nature's Cheat sheet**
     - Use this as a shopping guide to ensure your plate is as colourful and as nutritionally complete as possible. Aim for a Rainbow of food on your

plate and keep your fruits and vegetables as process-free as possible

- **Protein-Rich Breakfast Ideas**
    - A few ideas to get you started in the morning on the right track. Anyone of these ideas will help fuel your day, provide you with energy and optimal brain power
- **Homemade Bread Recipe**
    - Delicious, easy to make, and budget-friendly, this recipe will fill your home with one of the most pleasantly intoxicating smells known to man (freshly baked bread), while providing you with a stress-relieving activity (thanks to all that kneading), that you can do at night while de-electromagnetiying from the day's use of electronic devices.

7 Day Tracking Sheet

(You can download a printable version from my website: www.carlamjones.com/MemberResources) This tracking sheet gives you a glimpse of the *7 Day to a Healthier Happier You* program. As you can see below, each day has a new action step. This tracking sheet is applicable to Week 1 of the program.

In the weeks following the *7 Day to a Healthier Happier You* program, all of the actions listed on the left should be done every day. You can create your own tracking sheet, or purchase *"31 Days to a Healthier Happier You"* program (available in June 2015) for a full tracking sheet and daily routine schedule.

7 Day Tracking Sheet - Week 1

	MON	TUES	WED	THURS	FRI	SAT	SUN
Morning Lemon water	X	X	X	X	X	X	X
Water before lunch	optional but highly recommended						
Water before dinner	optional but highly recommended						

	MON	TUES	WED	THURS	FRI	SAT	SUN
7 Day Tracking Sheet - Week 1							
30mins no devices before bed		X	X	X	X	X	X
20 mins walking			X		X		X
whole food morning snack				X	X	X	X
whole foods at lunch				X	X	X	X
whole food afternoon snack				X	X	X	X
whole foods at dinner				X	X	X	X
10-15min of sun					X	X	X

7 Day Tracking Sheet - Week 1							
	MON	**TUES**	**WED**	**THURS**	**FRI**	**SAT**	**SUN**
Protein-rich breakfast						**X**	**X**
change negative self-talk							**X**

Nature's Cheat Sheet

(You can download a printable version from my website: www.carlamjones.com/MemberResources)

Nature's Cheat Sheet for our Wellbeing			
	Possible Health Benefits studied	**Vitamins and Nutrients**	**Examples of produce**
Orange / Yellow	• Boosts Immune system • Improves Vision health • Fights age-related macula degeneration • Lowers risk of prostate cancer • Lowers LDL (Bad) cholesterol • Lowers blood pressure • Promotes collagen formation • Healthy joints • Good for skin • Improves Bone health • Anti-inflammatory • Helps blood sugar regulation	• Antioxidants • Vitamin A • Vitamin C • Flavonoids • Lycopene • Potassium	Apricots, Butternut squash, Cantaloupe, Cape Gooseberries, Carrots, Golden kiwifruit, Grapefruit, Lemon, Mangoes, Nectarines, Oranges, Papayas, Peaches, Persimmons, Pineapples, Pumpkin, Rutabagas, Sweet corn, Sweet potatoes, Tangerines, Yellow apples, Yellow beets, Yellow figs, Yellow pears, Yellow peppers, Yellow potatoes, Yellow summer squash, Yellow tomatoes, Yellow watermelon, Yellow winter squash

Nature's Cheat Sheet for our Wellbeing

	Possible Health Benefits studied	Vitamins and Nutrients	Examples of produce
Blue / Purple	• Improves memory • Reduces disease risk by preventing clots • Improves blood pressure • Lowers risk of cancer in digestive tract • Limits activity of cancer cells • Supports retinal health • Lowers LDL (bad) cholesterol • Boosts immune system • Supports healthy digestion • Improves calcium and other mineral absorption • Anti-inflammatory	• Phytonut-rients (Antho-cyanins) • Lutein • Vitamin C • Fiber • Flavonoids • Ellagic acid • Quercetin	Black currants, Black salsify, Blackberries, Blueberries, Dried plums, Eggplant, Elderberries, Grapes, Plums, Pomegranates, Prunes, Purple Belgian endive, Purple Potatoes, Purple asparagus, Purple cabbage, Purple carrots, Purple figs, Purple grapes, Purple peppers, Raisins
Green	• Improves vision by supporting retinal health • Reduces risk of disease • Reduces carcinogenic compounds • Prevents blood clotting • Lowers blood pressure	• Chlorophyll • Fiber • Lutein • Calcium • Vitamin C • Folate • Vitamin K • Potassium • Carotenoids	Artichokes, Arugula, Asparagus, Avocados, Broccoflower, Broccoli, Broccoli rabe, Brussel sprouts, Celery, Chayote squash, Chinese cabbage, Cucumbers, Endive, Green apples,

Nature's Cheat Sheet for our Wellbeing

	Possible Health Benefits studied	Vitamins and Nutrients	Examples of produce
	• Reduces LDL (bad) cholesterol • Normalizes digestion time • Books immune system		Green beans, Green cabbage, Green grapes, Green onion, Green pears, Green peppers, Honeydew, Kiwifruit, Leafy greens, Leeks, Lettuce, Limes, Okra, Peas, Snow Peas, Spinach, Sugar snap peas, Watercress, Zucchini
Red	• Powerful antioxidant • Reduced risk of some cancers, • Protection against heart attacks • Lowers risk of prostate cancer • Fights bad bacteria • Lowers blood pressure • Reduces tumour growth • Lowers LDL (bad) Cholesterol • Supports joint tissue	• Lycopene • Anthocyanin • Vitamin C • Folate, • Flavonoids • Tannins • Ellagic acid	Beets, Blood oranges, Cherries, Cranberries, Guava, Papaya, Pink grapefruit, Pink/Red grapefruit, Pomegranates, Radicchio, Radishes, Raspberries, Red apples, Red bell peppers, Red chili peppers, Red grapes, Red onions, Red pears, Red peppers, Red potatoes, Rhubarb, Strawberries, Tomatoes, Watermelon

Nature's Cheat Sheet for our Wellbeing			
	Possible Health Benefits studied	Vitamins and Nutrients	Examples of produce
White	• Promotes Heart-Health • Reduces risk of disease • Powerful immune booster • Natural killer of B and T cells • Reduces risk of colon, breast and prostate cancers • Balances hormone levels • Reduces risk of hormone-related cancers	• Alicin • Beta-glucans	Bananas, Brown pears, Cauliflower, Dates, Garlic, Ginger, Jerusalem artickoke, Jicama, Kohlrabi, Mushrooms, Onions, Parsnips, Potatoes, Shallots, Turnips, White Corn, White nectarines, White peaches

Protein-Rich Breakfast ideas

- Oatmeal made with Almond milk, served with Almond butter, Banana, Maple syrup, Chia seeds and Flaxseeds
- Western Omelette (Cheese, tomato, onion, spinach)
- Homemade muesli served with whole fat Greek-Style unsweetened natural yoghurt (or, even better, Natural Goat's yoghurt)
- Poached Eggs, roasted Asparagus, wilted Spinach and Oat cakes
- Breakfast wrap with roasted Chicken breast, tomato, goat's cheese, beet greens
- Egg baked in an avocado cup (pitted avocado half) with side salad
- Scrambled eggs with onions, chives, Vegetables and Chia seeds
- Fruit and Nuts with Cottage Cheese (whole fat) and sprinkle of cinnamon
- Smoked salmon on Rye bread with Cottage cheese and a mix of berries on the side

You can always easily ramp up the protein intake of your breakfast by:

- Sprinkling flavourless whey protein powder
- Sprinkling Chia seeds, Flax seeds, Pumpkin Seeds, Sesame Seeds
- Adding nuts (Almonds, Cashews, Pecans, Walnuts, Brazil nuts etc)

Homemade Wholewheat Bread

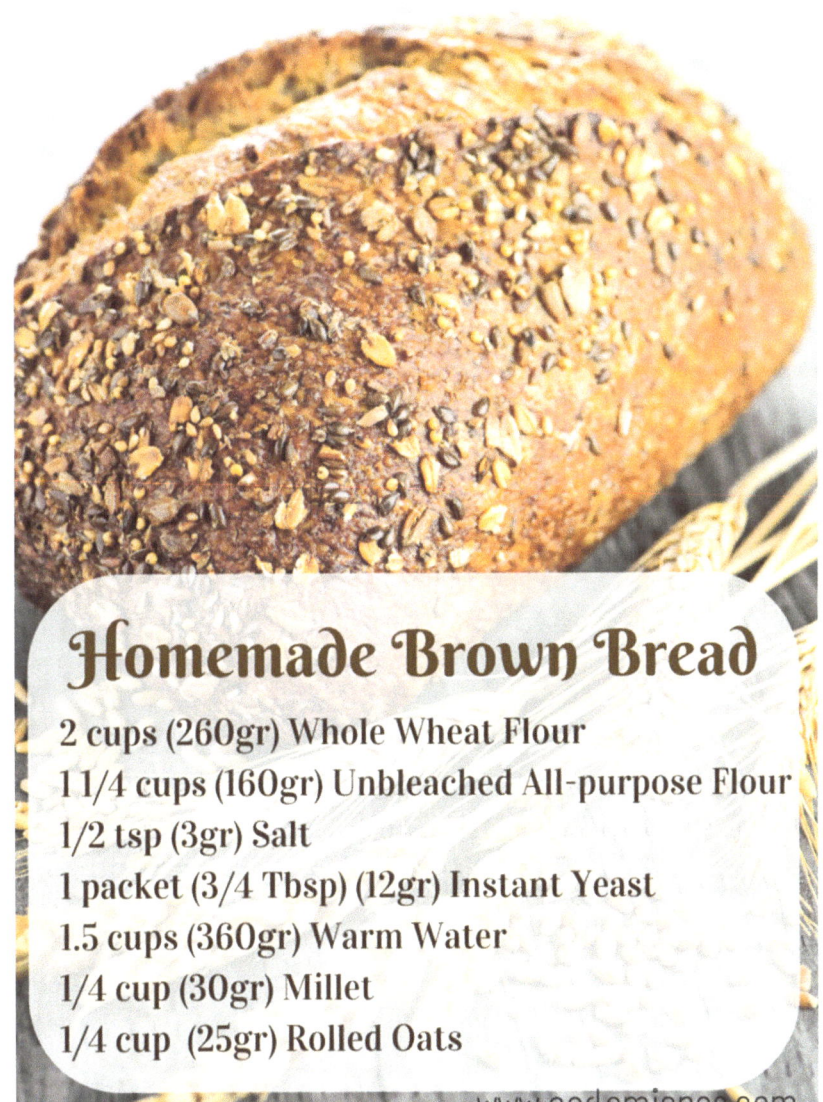

Homemade Brown Bread

2 cups (260gr) Whole Wheat Flour

1 1/4 cups (160gr) Unbleached All-purpose Flour

1/2 tsp (3gr) Salt

1 packet (3/4 Tbsp) (12gr) Instant Yeast

1.5 cups (360gr) Warm Water

1/4 cup (30gr) Millet

1/4 cup (25gr) Rolled Oats

www.carlamjones.com

Instructions

- Combine warm water with yeast in a a glass and let stand for 5 minutes to get foamy.
- In a large mixing bowl, mix the flours together. Make a well in the centre. Add the salt to one of the sides of the flower and pour the yeast mixture into the well (if the salt touches the yeast, it will kill it and the bread will not rise). Stir with a wooden spoon. The result will be a sticky, rough dough.
- Lift the dough out of the bowl and lightly grease the bowl with olive oil. Cover with plastic wrap and let rise in the in a warm place for 1 hour.
- Once doubled in size, lightly sprinkle the dough with flour and transfer to a generously floured work surface. Knead a few times adding flour as needed and then add oats and millet in batches. Knead until until grains are incorporated and the dough is no longer sticky. Knead with the palm of your hand pushing the dough away from you, bringing it back in, then pushing it away again. Do this until the dough is fairly smooth.
- Place on lightly greased baking sheet. Sift a light coating of flour over the top to help keep the dough moist. Let rest for 45-60 minutes in a warm place.
- Preheat oven to 450°F (230°C) and place a metal or cast iron pan (not glass, Pyrex, or ceramic) on the lowest oven rack, and have 1 cup of hot water ready. (If you have a steam oven, you do not require the pan on the bottom rack. Just follow your oven's

instructions on how to use steam when baking bread).

- When ready to bake, slash the bread 2 or 3 times with a knife, making a cut about ½-inch deep.
- Place bread in oven and carefully pour hot water into the shallow pan on the rack beneath. Close oven door quickly.
- Bake the bread for 25 to 35 minutes, or until golden brown and crusty. Knocking the bread on the bottom will sound hollow.
- Remove the bread from the oven and cool on a rack. Once fully cooled, store leftovers in a plastic bag at room temp.

This recipe has been adapted from:
www.minimalistbaker.com

ANYONE CAN GIVE UP
IT'S THE EASIEST THING
IN THE WORLD
TO DO
BUT TO HOLD IT TOGETHER
WHEN EVERYONE ELSE
WOULD UNDERSTAND
IF YOU FELL APART
THAT'S TRUE STRENGTH

www.carlamjones.com